THE PICTURE B

UNIVERSE

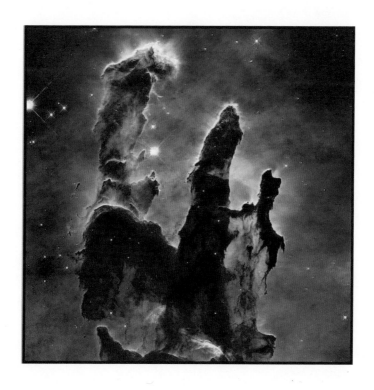

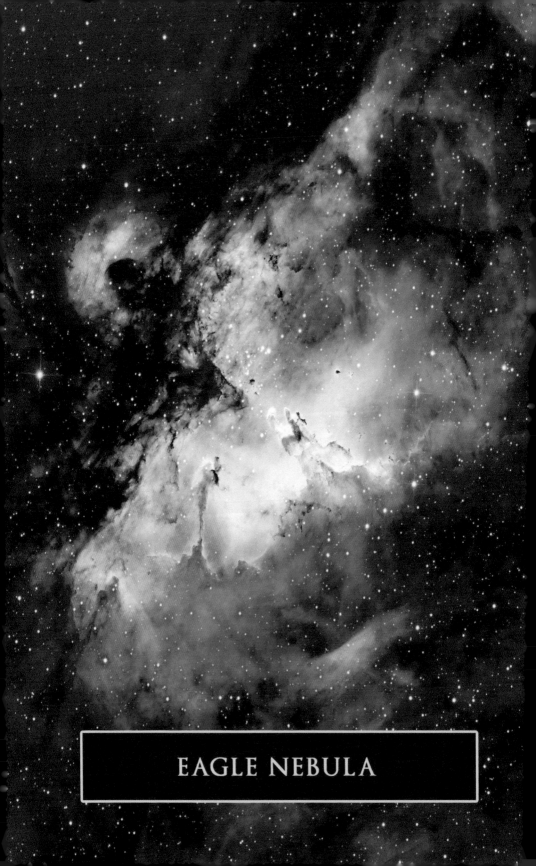

EAGLE NEBULA

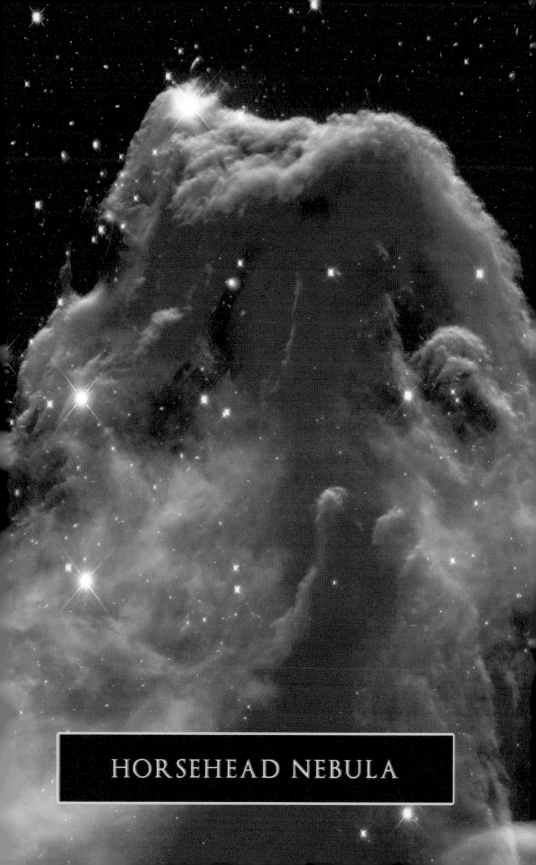

HORSEHEAD NEBULA

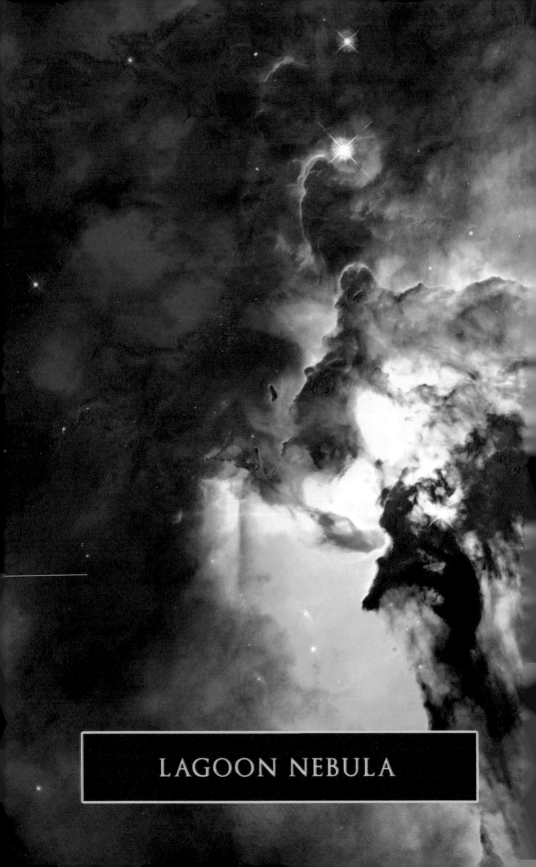

LAGOON NEBULA

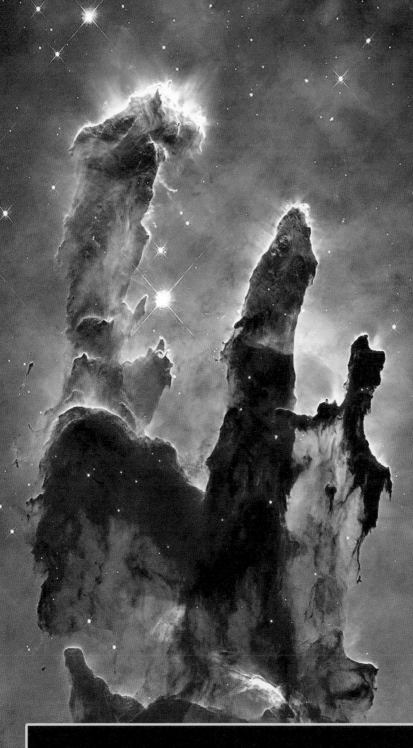

PILLARS OF CREATION

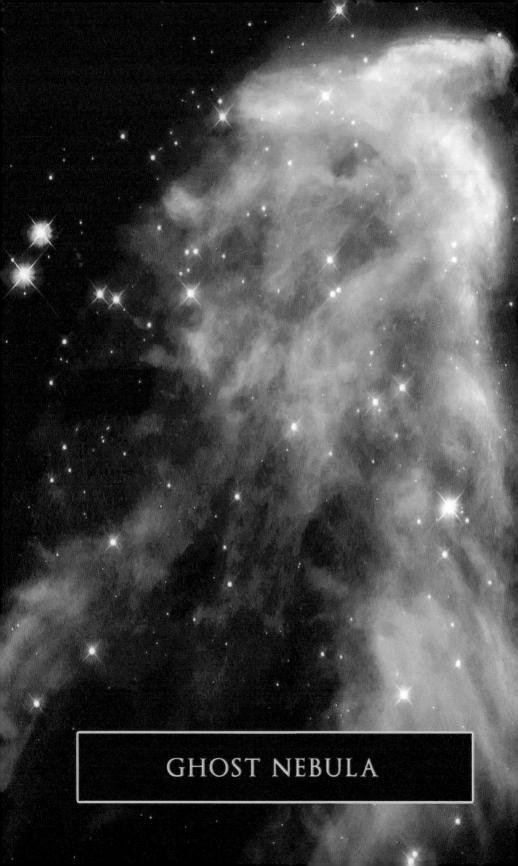

GHOST NEBULA

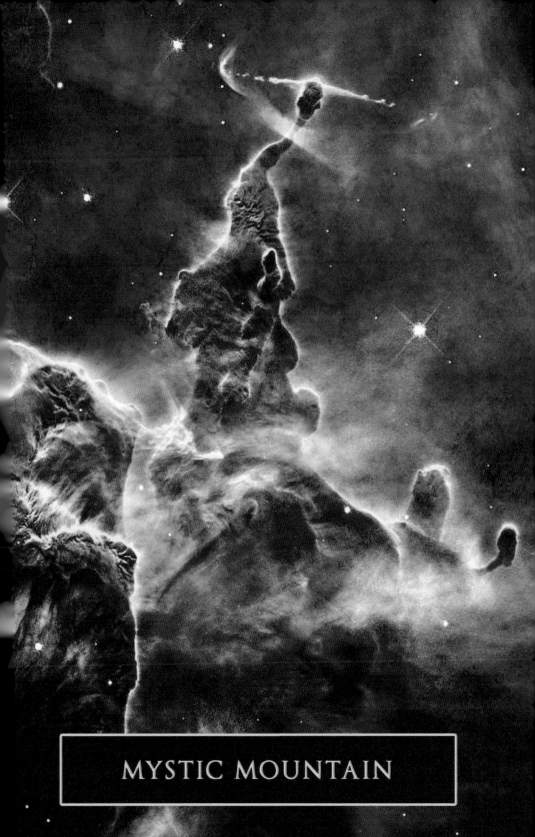

MYSTIC MOUNTAIN

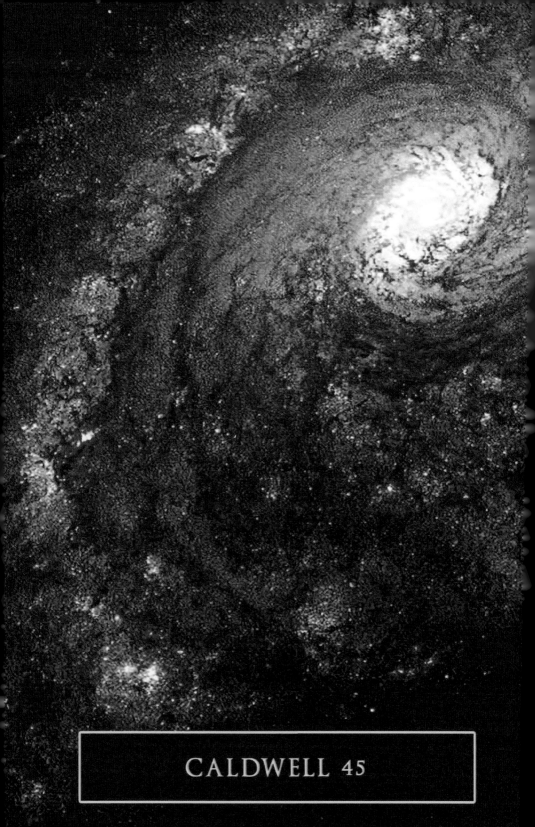

CALDWELL 45

DRAGONFISH NEBULA

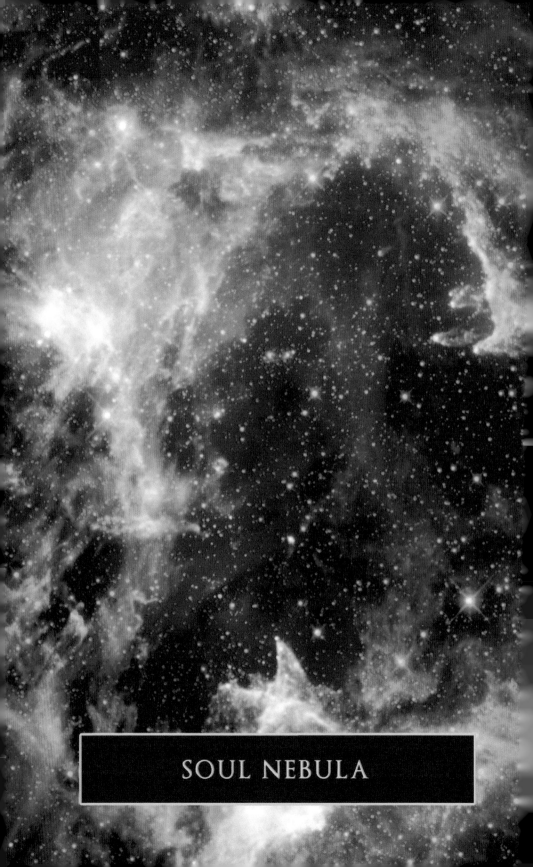

SOUL NEBULA

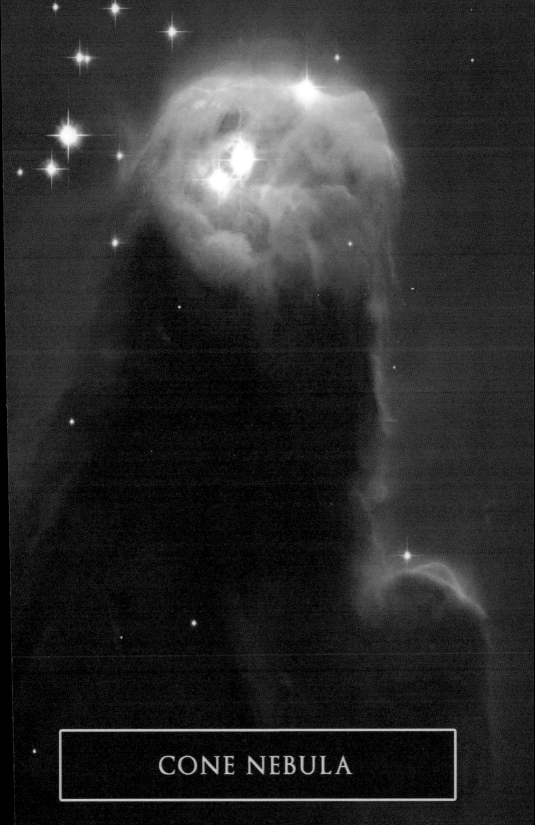

CONE NEBULA

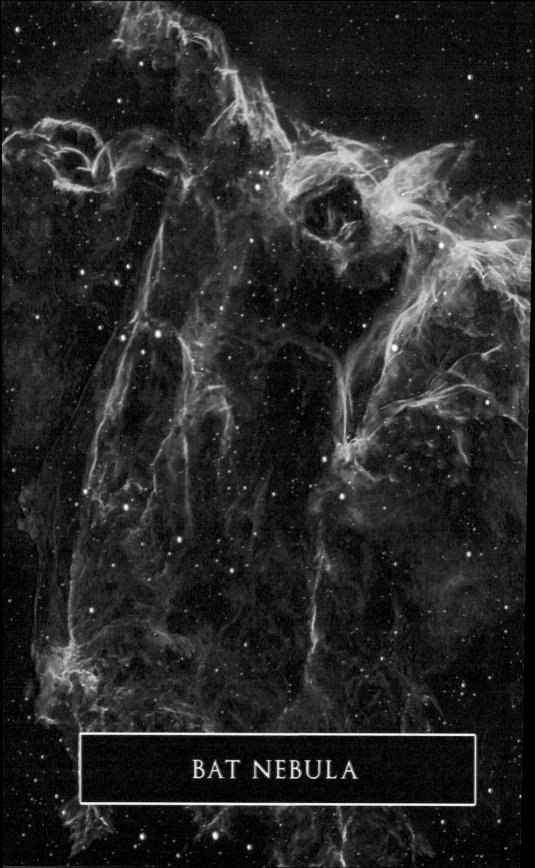

BAT NEBULA

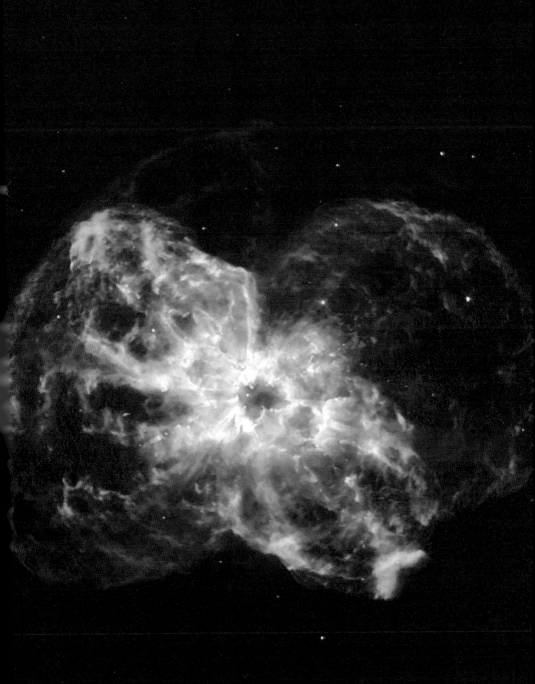

BOW TIE NEBULA

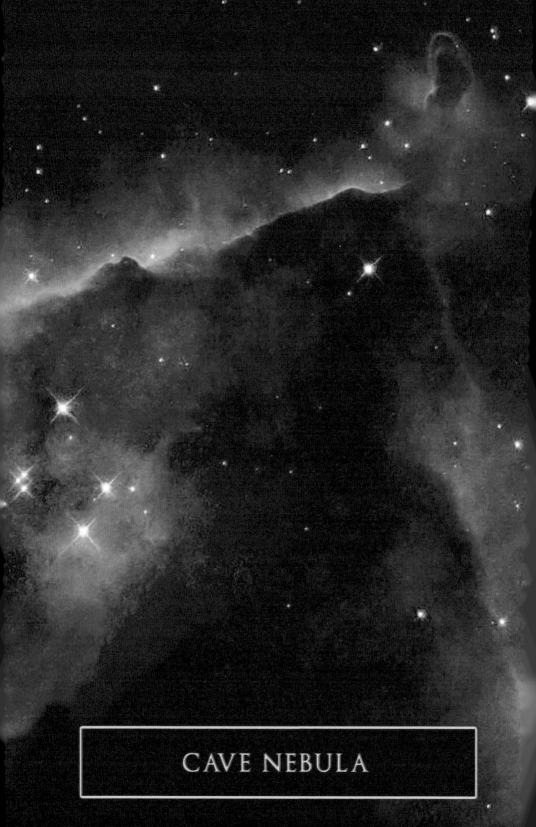

CAVE NEBULA

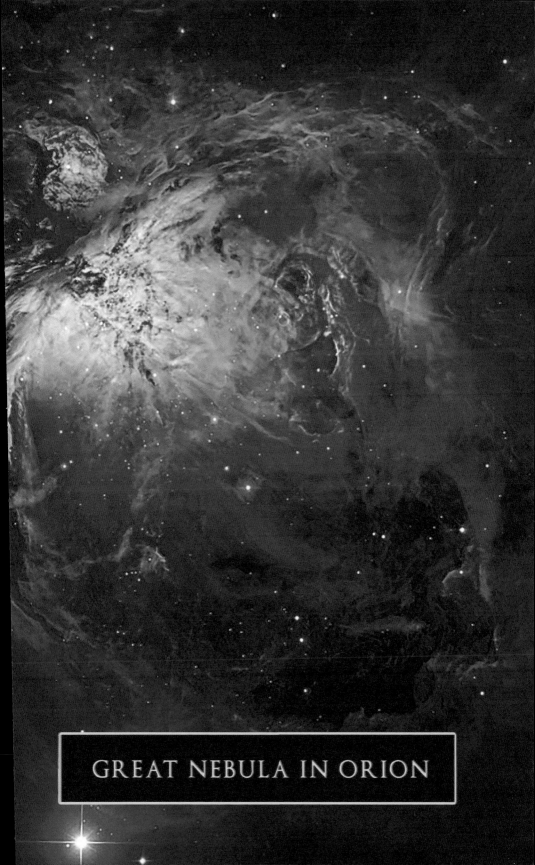

GREAT NEBULA IN ORION

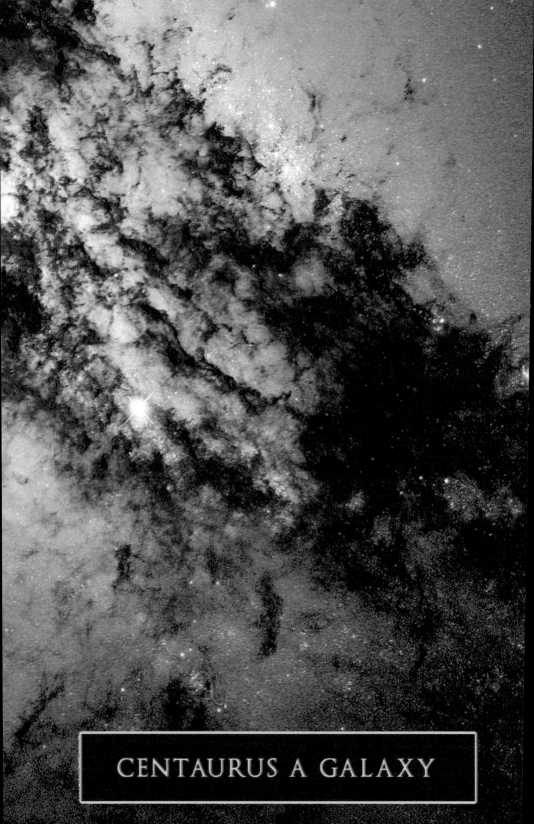

CENTAURUS A GALAXY

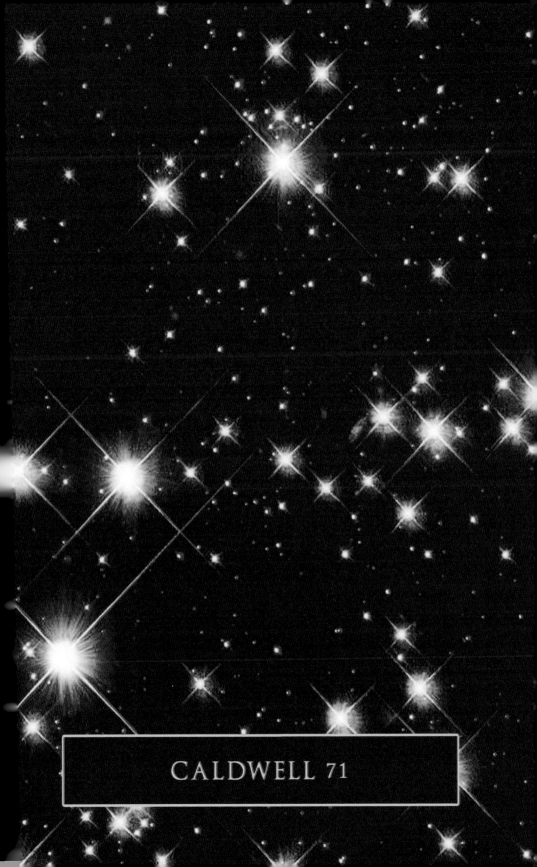

CALDWELL 71

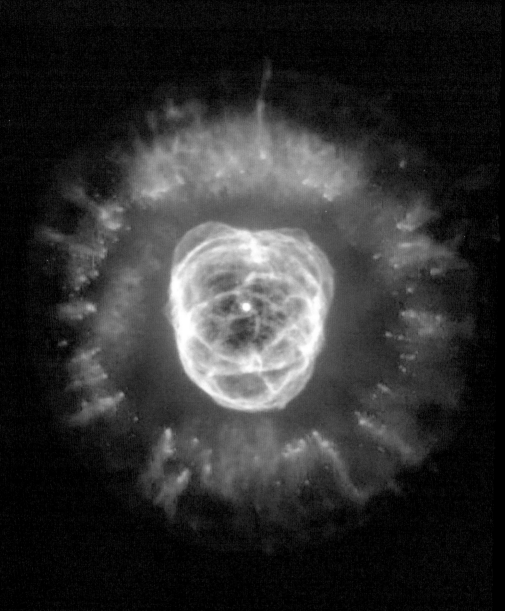

CALDWELL 39

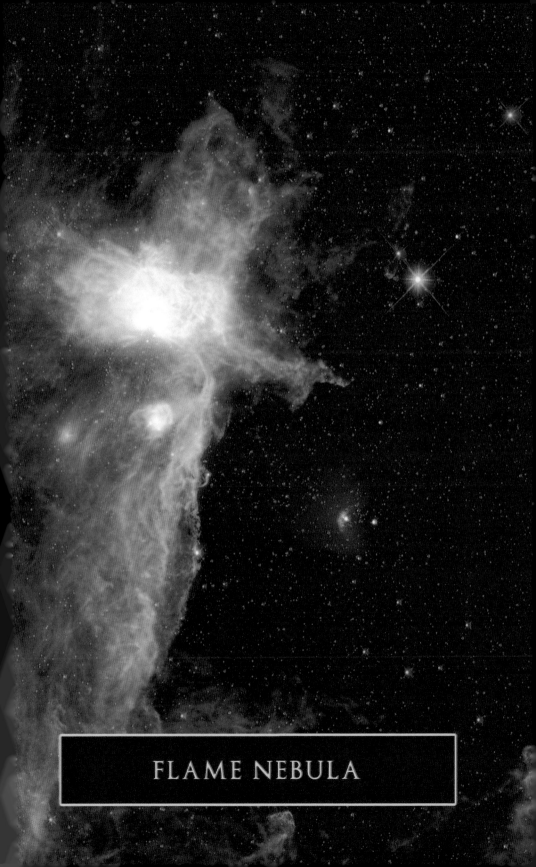

FLAME NEBULA

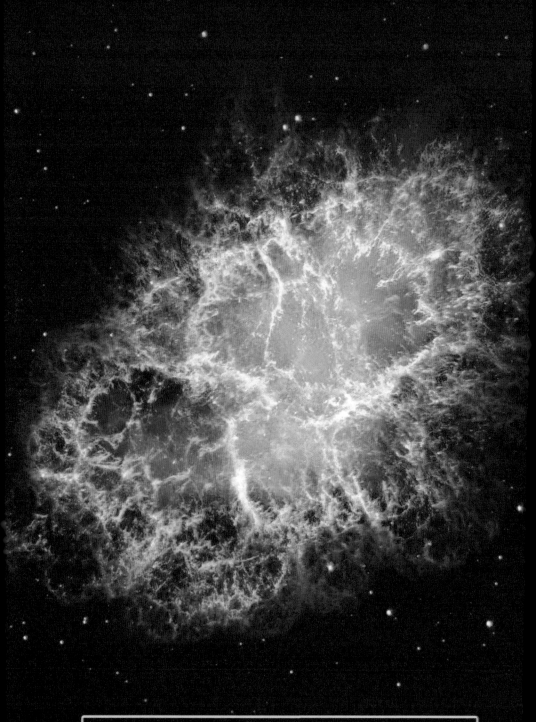

CRAB NEBULA

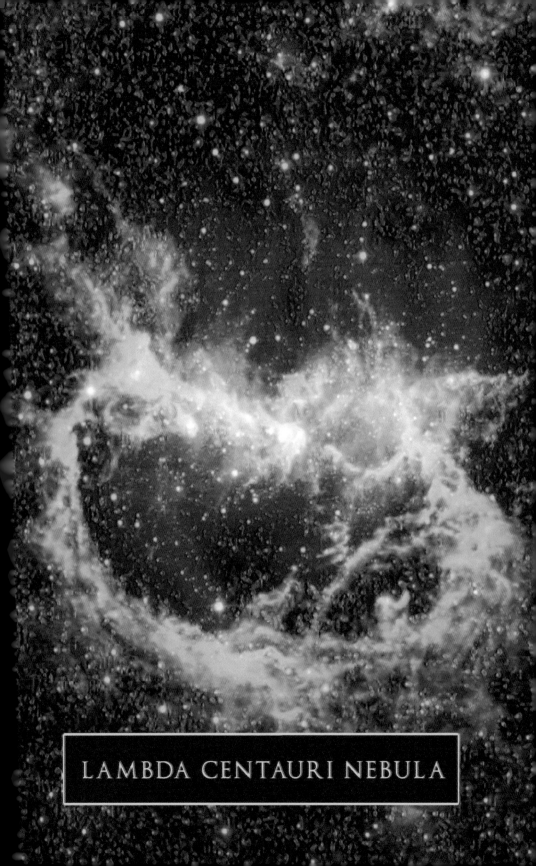

LAMBDA CENTAURI NEBULA

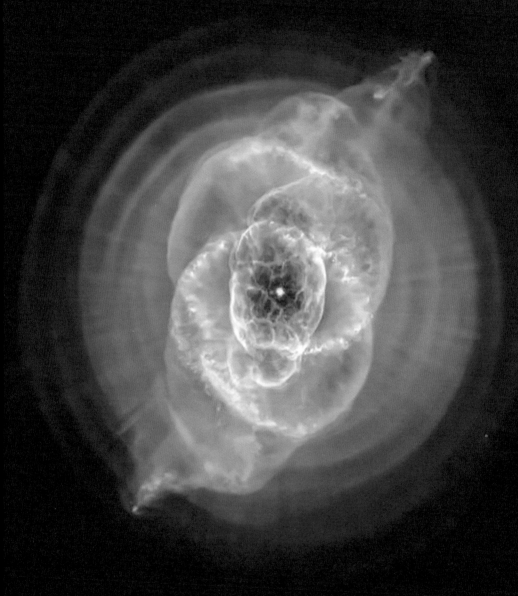

CAT'S EYE NEBULA

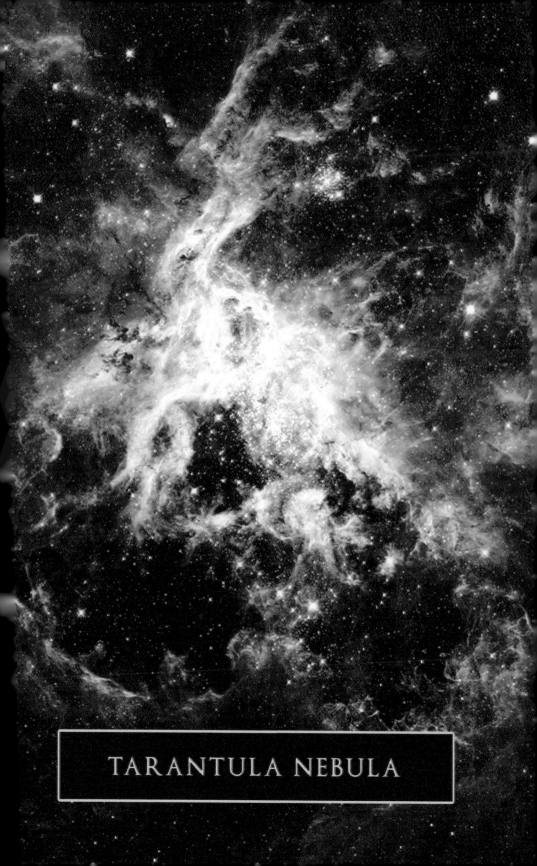

TARANTULA NEBULA

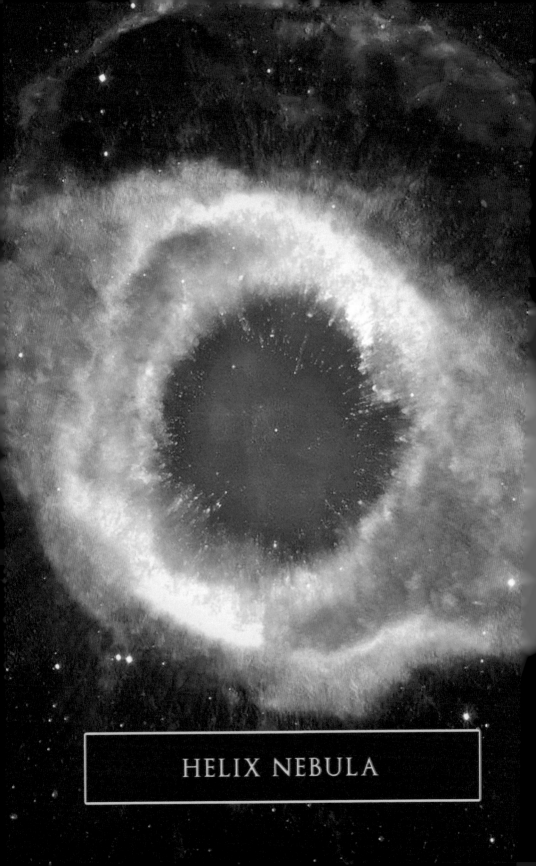

HELIX NEBULA

NORTH AMERICA NEBULA

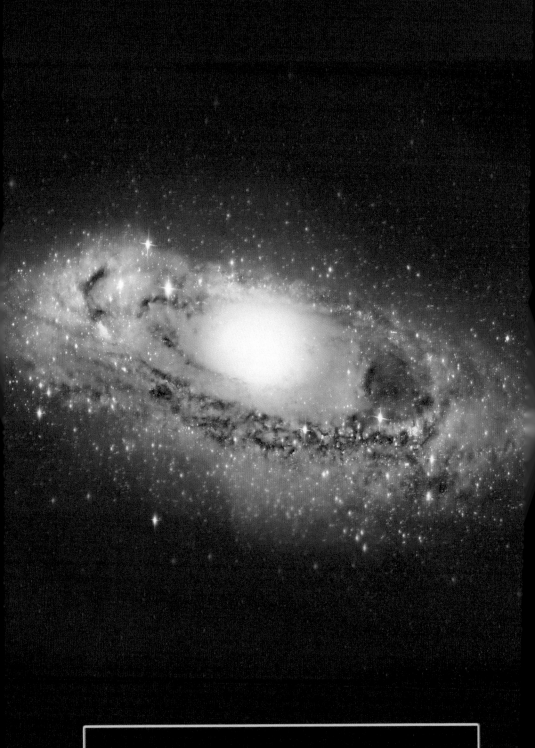

MILKY WAY GALAXY

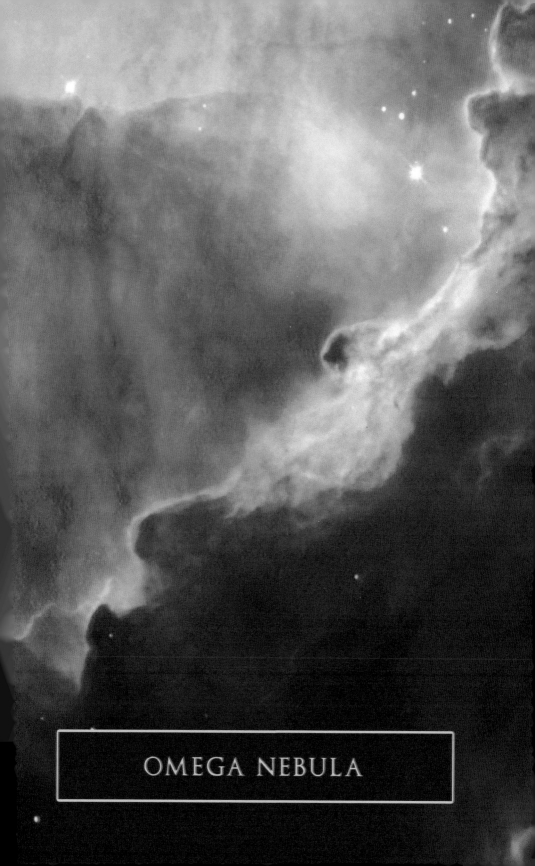

OMEGA NEBULA

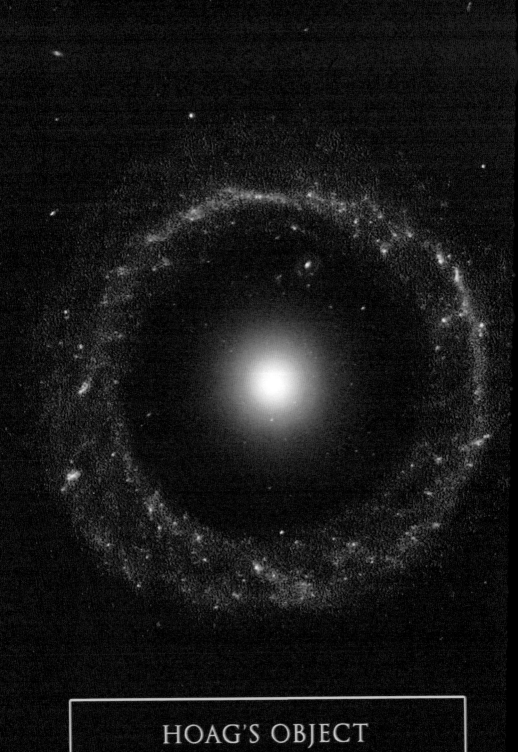

HOAG'S OBJECT

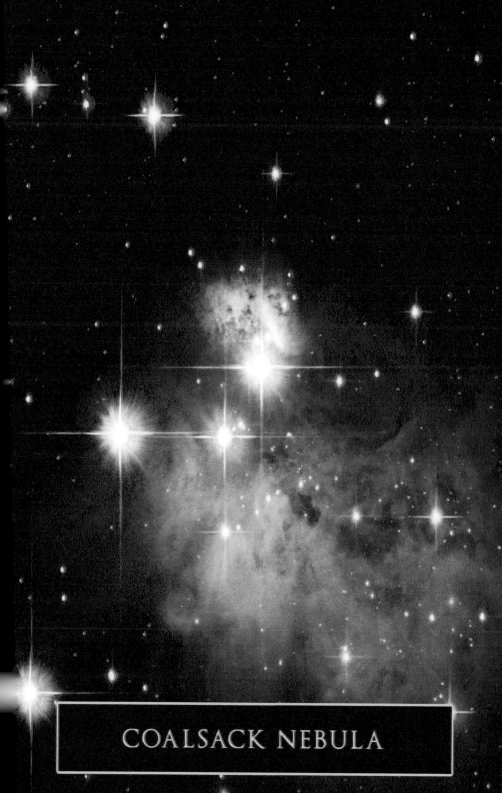

COALSACK NEBULA

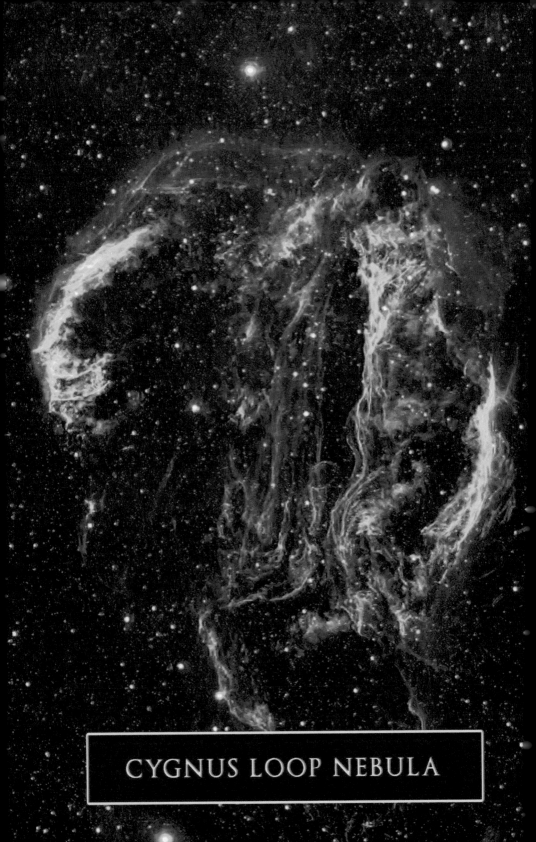

CYGNUS LOOP NEBULA

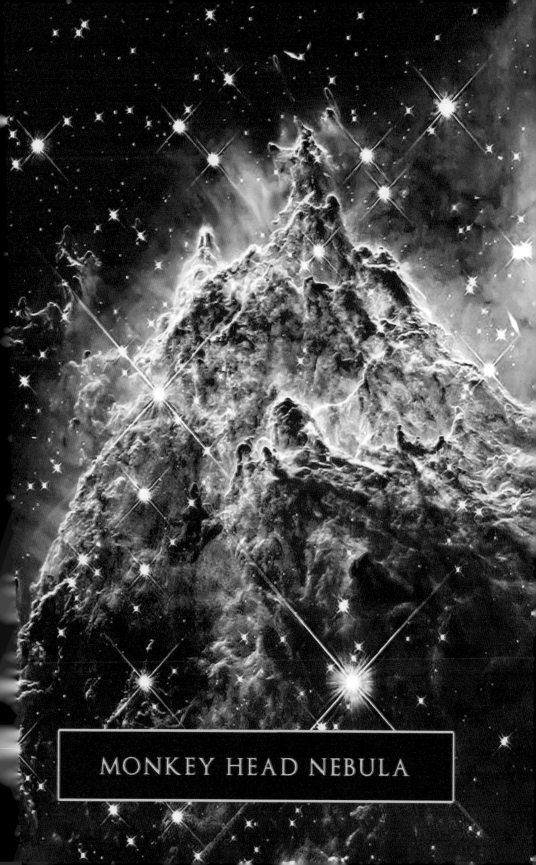

MONKEY HEAD NEBULA

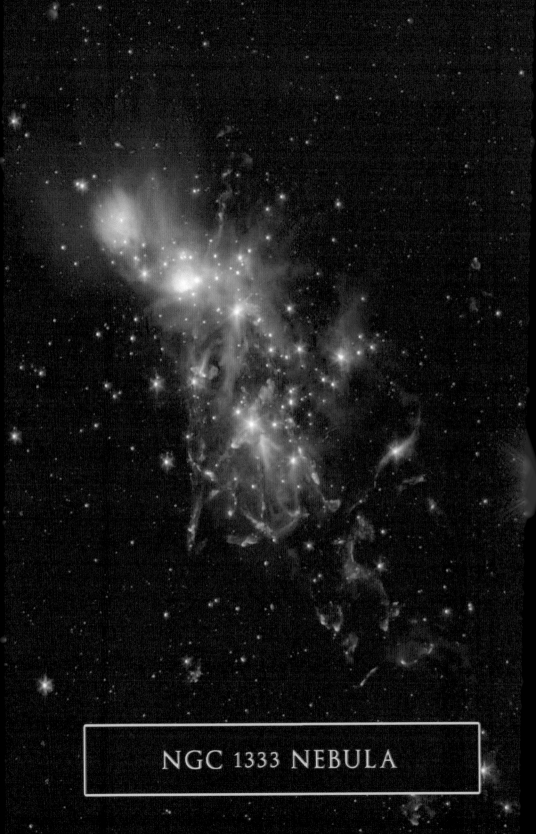

NGC 1333 NEBULA

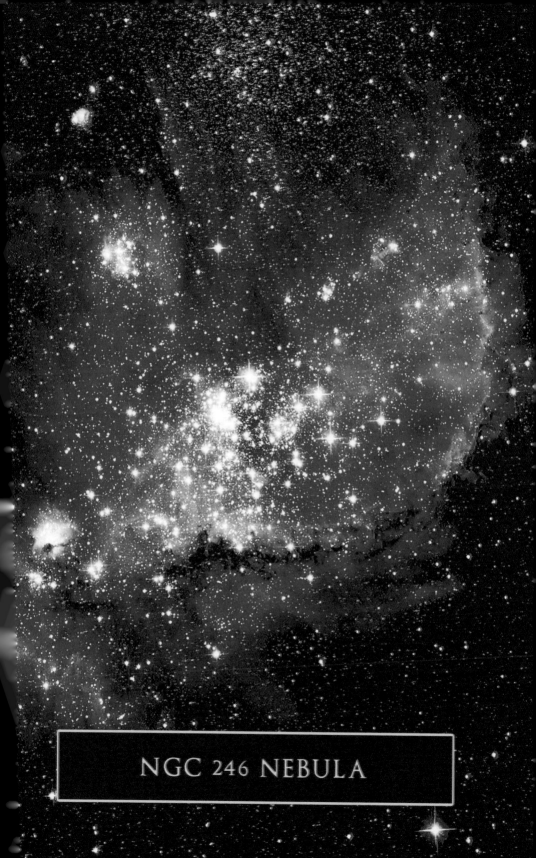

NGC 246 NEBULA

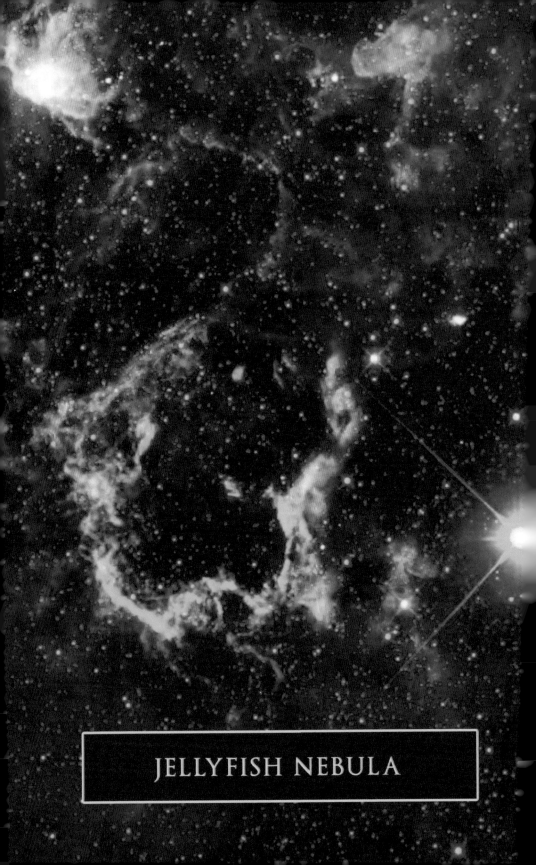

JELLYFISH NEBULA

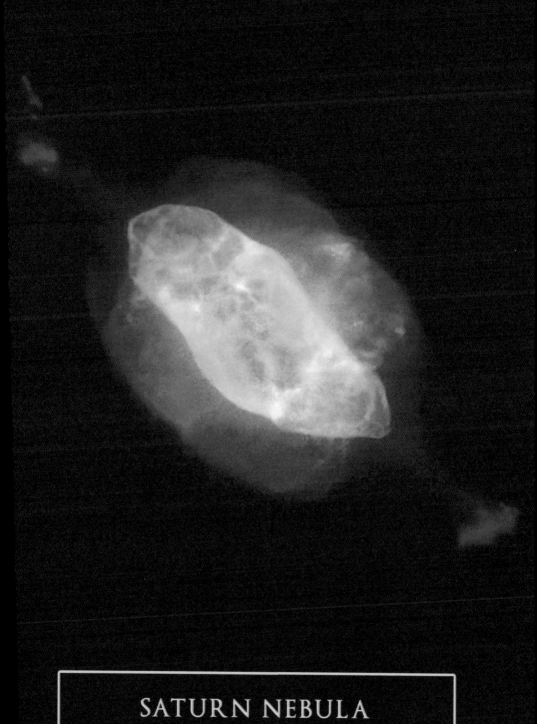

SATURN NEBULA

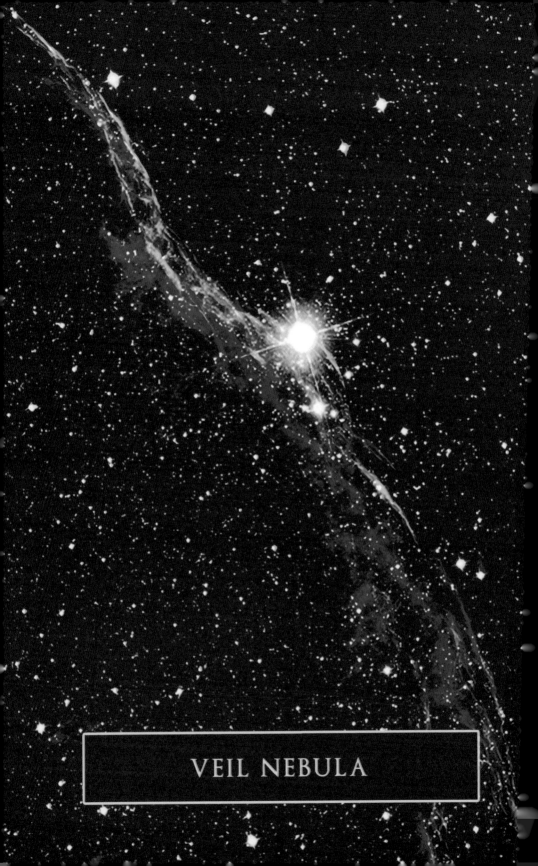

VEIL NEBULA

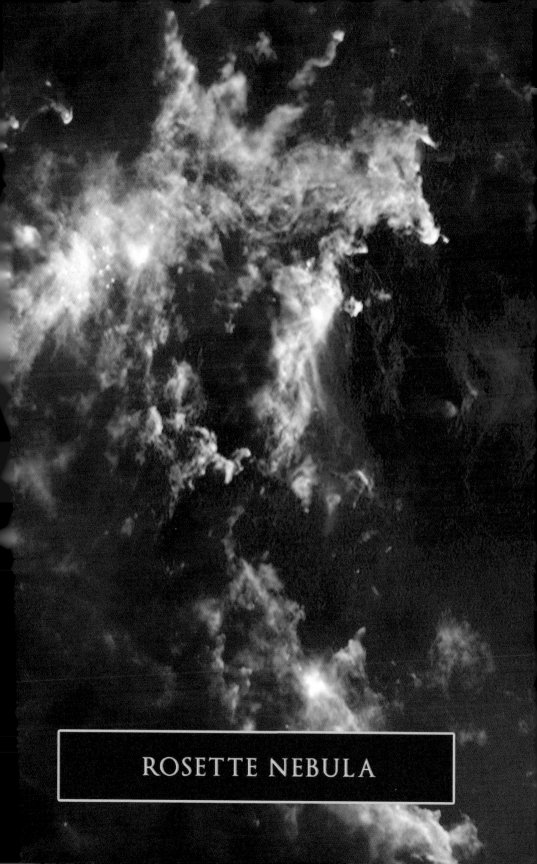

ROSETTE NEBULA

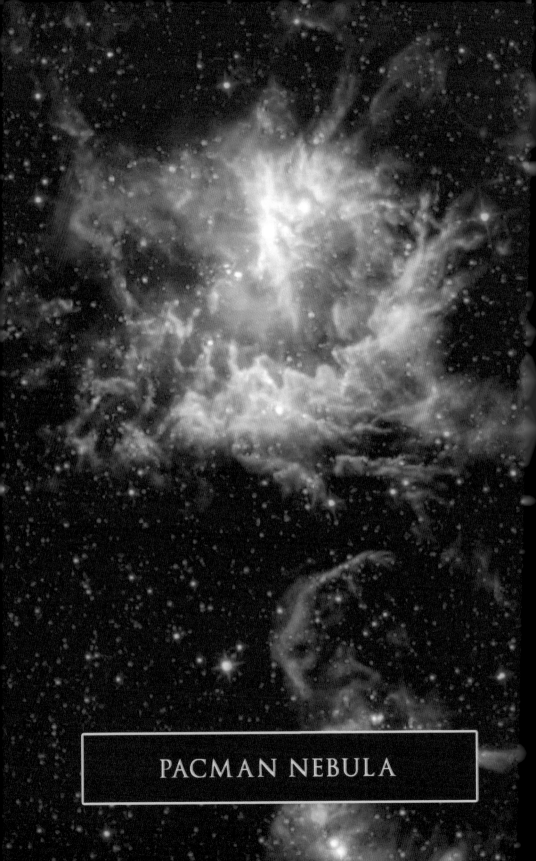

PACMAN NEBULA

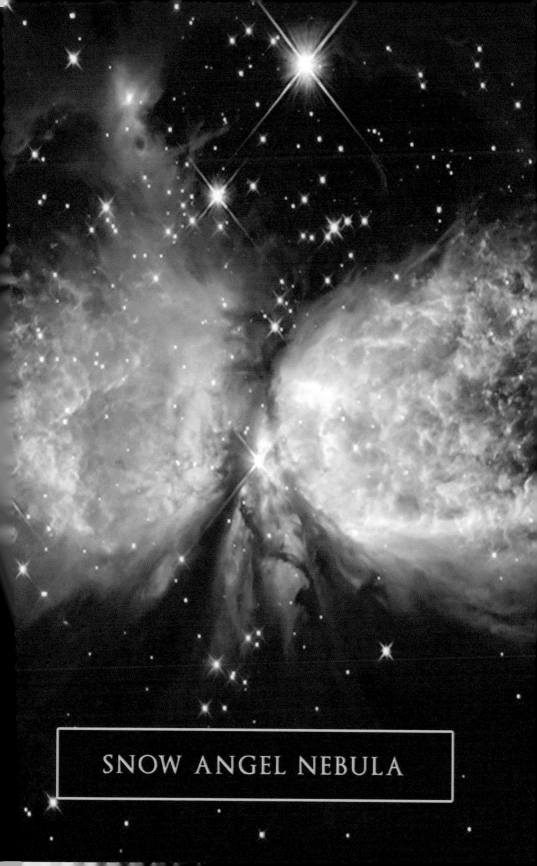

SNOW ANGEL NEBULA

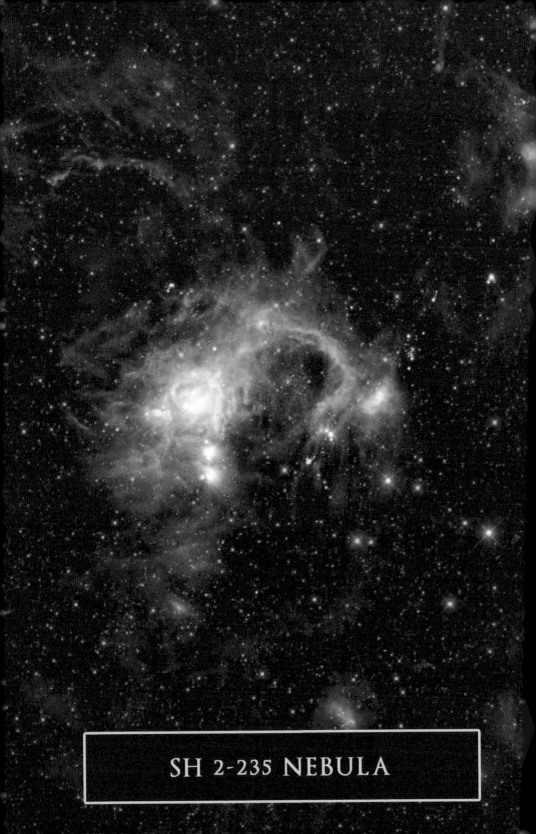

SH 2-235 NEBULA

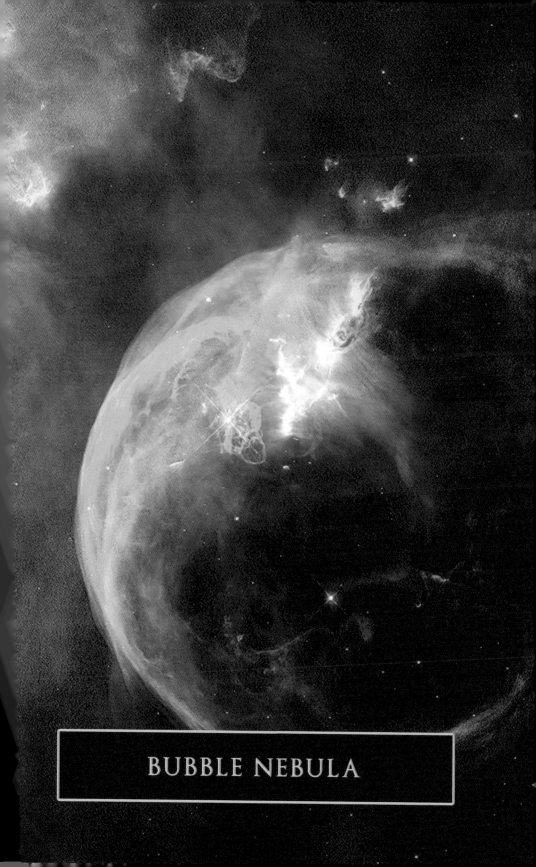

BUBBLE NEBULA

Printed in Great Britain
by Amazon

21960303R00025

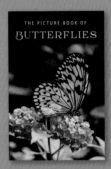
THE PICTURE BOOK OF
BUTTERFLIES

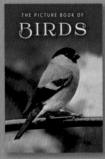
THE PICTURE BOOK OF
BIRDS

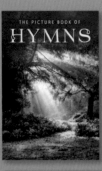
THE PICTURE BOOK OF
HYMNS

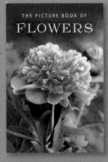
THE PICTURE BOOK OF
FLOWERS

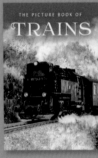
THE PICTURE BOOK OF
TRAINS

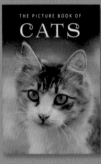
THE PICTURE BOOK OF
CATS

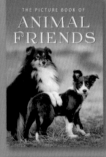
THE PICTURE BOOK OF
ANIMAL
FRIENDS

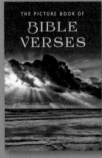
THE PICTURE BOOK OF
BIBLE
VERSES

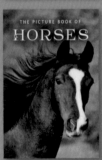
THE PICTURE BOOK OF
HORSES

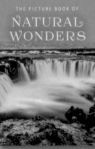
THE PICTURE BOOK OF
NATURAL
WONDERS

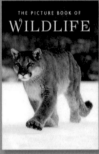
THE PICTURE BOOK OF
WILDLIFE

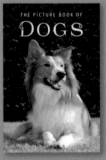
THE PICTURE BOOK OF
DOGS

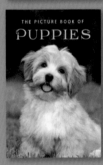
THE PICTURE BOOK OF
PUPPIES

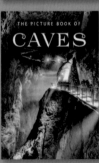
THE PICTURE BOOK OF
CAVES

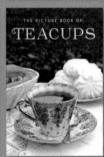
THE PICTURE BOOK OF
TEACUPS

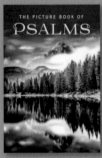
THE PICTURE BOOK OF
PSALMS

SUNNY STREET
BOOKS

SunnyStreetBooks.com

ISBN 9798588259415

9000

9 798588 259415

DESIGN
YOUR OWN WEBSITE
WITH WORDPRESS
2023

The ultimate, step-by-step, beginner's guide
to a full-featured WordPress website
for small business, coaches, authors & bloggers

NO CODING REQUIRED | SAVE EXPENSIVE DESIGNER FEES

NARAYAN KUMAR